MOM'S NATURAL SOLUTION TO EVERYDAY LIVING

Lorraine S Shikapwashya

ISBN: 1496162587
ISBN 13: 9781496162588

CONTENTS

DEDICATION

To my God who has walked with me and is my strength every day.

To my husband Aiza for his love, support and encouragement.

To my children Gabriella, A.J and Adriyel, thank you for your unconditional love and teaching me to enjoy the simple things in life.

To my Mother Rita who has overcome a lot of hardship in life yet she continues to smile, thanks for loving me.

ACKNOWLEDGEMENTS

A special thanks to Wendy Holibough, Ms Beth Duncan, Pastor Russell Hodgins, Pastor and Mrs. Stan Siwek, my church family at Westchester Christian Worship Center, my siblings Yvonne, Helen(late), Nyasha(late), Mona(late), Emmanuel, Susan and Michael, Herta and my numerous friends . Thank you for your encouragement, love and support. I am truly grateful. May God bless you all.

INTRODUCTION

I remember driving to the pharmacy to pick up a prescription for my son after a sick visit to his pediatrician. It was past mid day, I had three hungry children in the back of the car under the age of five and our plans for that day had gone out through the window. It almost felt like this had become a theme in our lives. Should common childhood ailments be this common? What if there is something I can do to promote the health of my children to avoid them? It is these thoughts that started it all.

Over the past six years, I have been on an extraordinary and revealing journey where I began to learn and slowly to make changes that promote my family's health. The more I learned, the more I was inspired. The small changes were yielding big results. These enlightening paths stirred a passion within me to share what I learned with moms who, like myself, juggle priorities, make sacrifices, and sometimes just try to make it one day at a time in "Mommyville." My belief is that, although the details of our lives as women may differ, the common thread of our motherhood unites us.

Mom's Natural Solution to Everyday Living is an attempt to help mothers who sincerely want the best for their families. It is an effort to sound the alarm of the hidden and harmful effects of chemicals found in everyday products and to offer more natural and healthier alternatives. The toxic compounds that come into our homes in the form of convenient goods such as plastic make our lives easier but unhealthier over time due to constant exposure.

It is my prayer that after reading this book, you will become more alert and aware and will start a more informed conversation with other moms about their choices as selective and educated consumers. Most importantly it is my hope that women would no longer make purchases based on price, brand, or appeal, but on a product's quality. The extra attention to detail while shopping is no longer a privilege but a necessity. Your family is worth it.

WHY GREEN AND NATURAL SOLUTIONS ARE BEST

My journey to seek a healthier life has taken me through many paths, and one of those paths was choosing to embrace a "greener" lifestyle. "Going green" means taking steps toward a life that promotes health, happiness, and family time, while choosing to reduce my ecological impact on our planet.

My goal never has been to be perfect ecologically because no one is perfect. I realized, however, that I needed to be aware of my impact on not only the earth but also on my family that depended on me. If I was making mistakes that could cost my family their health, I knew there must be many other moms who were unaware of these dangers lurking in our daily environments or even inside our homes. I am referring to *moms* throughout because they are usually the primary caregivers, although this is certainly not the case in every home. My desire is to encourage you, the reader, to be aware and equipped as you safeguard the health of your precious family.

As our world continues to evolve and the demands of society increase, science searches for ways to make our lives easier and more convenient. Although we should seek solutions that simplify our lives by changing the time-consuming methods of years past, the problem comes when the quality of goods is compromised and actually becomes dangerous. Even more concerning is when we unwittingly go along with these changes because our lives are so busy and sometimes distracted by the overload of media information everywhere we turn.

How many times do you go to the supermarket not with the intent of simply satisfying your shopping list but with equal consideration about the quality of food and products you are buying? Have we considered questions such as: What has gone into producing this product? Are they in their simplest form for the benefit of my body? What is the best detergent for my family based on the level of potentially harmful ingredients contained versus which detergent is the most effective?

Let us not forget the weekly sale at the supermarket. Are you excited about getting a bargain based solely on the quantity rather than the nutritional quality of a food? Where is the emphasis on the quality of our selections? These questions are a great starting point; they will serve to get us to a place where we begin to analyze our thinking and ultimately to cause us to make the most informed healthy choices for our families.

We want to clean our houses quickly and easily without a lot of elbow grease. Today, unfortunately, that means chemicals are needed to get the job done easily, and we overlook the immediate and long-term exposure risks to our health, our children, pets, and the environment we live in. We would rather take nutritional supplements and microwave a store-bought meal than pour our energy into preparing meals made from real food prepared on the stove.

We need to think about what we are doing to ourselves and to our children. What kind of future are we creating for our children's children? *"It is a wise man who plants a tree in the shade of which he knows he will never sit."*—Greek Proverb. It is true that our diet and environment has evolved over time; equally true is that preventable childhood diseases such as obesity and juvenile diabetes have been on the rise in recent years, according to the Centers for Disease Control and Prevention. It is now being said that for the first time in history, this generation of children may not outlive their parents due to the obesity epidemic. Pat Waniewski, Director of the Health Department Bureau of Community Chronic disease Prevention shared this in 2012 at a presentation. Diseases such as childhood leukemia, brain cancer, asthma and attention deficit hyperactivity disorder, ADHD have been on the rise. Some have been linked to use of the pesticides, solvents and other toxins in the environment. According to the National Academy of Sciences, environmental factors contribute to over twenty eight percent of developmental disorders in children. We need to ensure that our children are protected from factors that predispose them to these diseases, whether at school or at home. For example asthma cases have increased tremendously resulting in frequent hospitalizations and school absenteeism not to mention the billions of dollars that are being spent in managing these cases. In fact researchers at Mount Sinai Hospital in New York were promoted to ask elected officials to step in and make some environmental changes to protect our children from these diseases. Thankfully the elected officials agreed with the scientists based on the evidence and plans are underway starting with a section of Harlem in New York City.

It is estimated that, in New York alone, children are exposed to more than eighty thousand different synthetic materials. Shockingly, nearly 80 percent of those chemicals have not been tested for their effects on humans. Our children are being exposed to chemicals that could very well be killing them, and nobody seems to be taking notice. It is up to you to stand up and advocate for your children. You must take it upon yourself to learn about the dangers and do as much as you can to limit the exposure to your children. I am not suggesting that you can avoid all harmful chemical exposure nor am I suggesting that you can save the world, but you certainly can take simple steps to reduce the amount of exposure. Even if you can't control all the dangers your children will be exposed to, by taking responsibility for the chemicals you allow into your home you will be making a difference in your family's health, even possibly lowering their risk for cancer. According to the American Cancer Society, cancer remains the second most common cause of death in the United States, accounting for nearly one of every four deaths. My prayer is that you will be stirred to analyze future purchases with an informed opinion. Throughout this book, you will discover the little things you can do in your home to make a positive change.

One easy fix is to spend a little more on organic produce, though organic foods may not look as perfect as conventional fruits and vegetables. Bigger may not always be better after all. Fruits and vegetables that are massive and perfect in color are usually the work of chemicals. There is nothing wrong with enjoying a typical tomato in all its natural glory without worrying about its size; generations before us thrived on these foods. There is a children's story that tells of a little boy who always wanted the biggest and best-looking everything his eyes fell upon. One day his mom taught him that bigger is not always better, and he soon discovered that the biggest pie was actually hollow on the inside. So it is with some of the food we buy in grocery stores that are big and beautiful. The awful truth is that they lack necessary nutrients and are full of toxins we do not want in the bodies of our growing Children. Childhood cancer for example has been linked to Pesticides used on food crops among other chemicals in the environment. It is time to go back to some of the more traditional ways of eating, gardening, and cleaning. There is a tremendous benefit of eating whole food that nourishes and boosts the body's immunity against diseases. Learning to rely on green and natural solutions is the best option for yourself and your family. This is not to suggest that you purchase everything that says *green* or *natural*, because there are many misleading labels.

You will want to know you are doing everything in your power to keep your family safe and healthy. Sure, it may take a little more work, but isn't your family worth it? It is more gratifying to know that you provide unadulterated food that promotes good health than resign to the alluring convenience while unconsciously harming your children with the food you are feeding them.

Green living isn't anything new, but it is a trend that is catching on, and people from all walks of life are realizing the benefits of eating a healthy diet and using safer products. The great news is that there are many resources to tap that will help with your new lifestyle, and the big plus is that there is competitive pricing on the goods and services you'll want when you transition to a greener way of living as many companies are beginning to offer more natural alternatives. Advocacy has played a big role in facilitating this shift.

One of the main reasons people continue to use dangerous cleaning products and eat unhealthy food is because they don't know any other way. Once you know alternatives to chemical-laden products, you can make informed decisions the next time you are in the store. The transition may seem intimidating, but the challenge is worth it for the sake of your family and the people you care about. I assure you, you will not be left with a dirty house because you shun products that you once considered good. Hopefully there will be a shift of the consumer mindset that you have toward food, personal care products, and cleaning products that you use every day. They will now have to be deemed safe based on your knowledge before you purchase them. Your home, your body, and your children's bodies will be just as clean, but without all the harmful chemicals. Sometimes your purchasing decisions will come down to evaluating which option is the lesser of two evils, and that's fine as long as you are making the best choice for your family.

NUTRITION

Over three hundred years ago wise words were spoken by the father of medicine Hippocrates when he said "Let food be thy medicine and medicine thy food."One of the most important aspects of everyday living is taking care of our bodies. As with anything we attempt to change, consistency is a key component of the process. Controlling what we put into our bodies on a regular basis will affect our health. Our bodies were designed to run like well-oiled machines. We can destroy the inner workings of our beautiful bodies, however, by putting things into them that will harm us. What we put in our bodies is absolutely crucial to our overall health. It isn't about just what tastes or smells good and is the easiest to grab; it is about what foods will help our body thrive. A healthy diet promotes good health and curbs the preventable diseases currently plaguing our society. There are several studies that suggest that with the right lifestyle, longevity may be attained. Chances are that you may live up to a decade longer. One such study is the Framingham heart study. Desiring longevity with vitality should be the ultimate goal.

THE PROBLEM

As a mom, if you do not read labels and you are not sure about what you need to look out for, it will be difficult to purchase wholesome food for your family. While it is tedious in the beginning, once you do it a few times, you will learn what to invest in for the long-term health of your family.

There is a strong emphasis in our society on the amount of calories, sugar, fat, and sodium in our food. Advocacy has resulted in the requirement of calorie counts to be displayed next to menu items. While I appreciate this change, when it comes to the overall quality of our food, this is not enough. The standard American diet corresponds to about eighteen to twenty-six teaspoons of extra sugar a day, based on a 1,800 to 2,600 calorie diet. Excessive sugar in your diet will not only make you gain weight but also weakens your immune system, leading to diabetes and other chronic diseases. The best known sugars are fructose ("fruit sugar") and sucrose ("table sugar"), but they are listed by other names as well: honey, dextrose, fructose, corn syrup, high-fructose corn syrup, sorbitol, fruit juice concentrate, galactose, lactose, polydextrose, mannitol, sorbitol, xylitol, maltodextrin, and turbinado. What is even more bizarre is to discover that, apart from the obvious offenders like soft drinks, candies, and other processed desserts, some savory foods such as salad dressing, protein bars, peanut butter, ketchup, tomato sauce, fast food, granola, canned soup, and bread have sugars in them that add to your daily sugar intake unbeknown to the consumer.

According to a November 6, 2013, CNN report, Kraft has agreed to stop producing children's macaroni and cheese with yellow dyes, namely yellow no. 5 and yellow no. 6. This is due to pressure from a blogger who sounded the alarm on this issue. Yellow no. 5 has been linked to hyperactivity, asthma, cancer, and other conditions.

Another recent development in the news as of February 2014 is that New York Senator Chuck Schumer called on the Food and Drug Administration to ban the use of the chemical azodicarbonamide in bread. It is used in as an additive and also used in one form in rubber products such as yoga mats and rubber soles for shoes. Once again a blogger was instrumental in sounding the alarm, which resulted in the recent decision by

Subway restaurant to remove the chemical from their breads. This chemical has been linked to cancer and asthma. These current and very public examples serve as a reminder that consumers must be vigilant about the food they consume but also that there is power in the individual's choices that can change food policy nationwide.

Foods that have been grown without the use of pesticides or chemical fertilizers are always the best bet. All of those chemicals sprayed on the plants to make them bigger and prettier are not always better. Where do all those chemicals go? They are absorbed into your blood, your brain, and your digestive system. Your children's little bodies are being exposed to these harsh chemicals at an early age. There really isn't a big secret as to why so many children are suffering from illnesses that were once reserved for adults and the elderly. Sadly, many of these ailments could be prevented by choosing not to pollute our children's bodies with things we know are toxic.

THE SOLUTION

Whenever possible, strive to eat whole foods with your family. Whole foods can be classified as those that are in their natural state and have not been processed or treated with unnatural chemical preservatives. These include food such as raw fruits, vegetables, nuts, grains, grass-fed animals, and free-range birds to name but a few. Sure, you can cook them yourself to change things up, but cook them in a way that preserves as much of the nutrients as possible. The most important thing to remember is that there will be some kind of nutrient degradation during storage and preparation. Simple things like buying local fresh, firm, crisp, unbruised fruit and vegetables which have not spent a week being shipped helps, avoid soaking chopped vegetables in water for a long time, steaming vegetables is better than boiling, if you do boil use the liquid as a broth. Over cooking food should be avoided as much as possible, reserve and use leafy greens as they have high concentrations of nutrients. The nutrients are what keep your body healthy. What many people don't realize is that the peel of a fruit and vegetable is often where the most nutrients are located, including beneficial enzymes. Think twice before you peel that apple or potato. Fresh food is always the best!

Meat such as skinless chicken breast is also much healthier than processed meat such as chicken nuggets. Busy moms certainly appreciate the convenience of those frozen foods that can be quickly popped in the microwave, but they are not good for the kids.

One trick you can use to save yourself some time during the week while keeping the kids happy is to prepare some homemade chicken nuggets ahead of time. This method is actually much less expensive than buying those premade nuggets that are filled with various byproducts and preservatives, not to mention lacking in significant nutritional value. Cook up a whole chicken or a pack of chicken breasts, and divide the meat into smaller, finger-sized pieces. Season them with your favorite spices and bake. Store the chicken in an airtight container, and pop it in the freezer. When you are in a hurry and need a quick lunch for the kids, pull out the chicken, heat it up, and you have a healthy alternative to heavily processed chicken nuggets.

Do not forget the benefit and convenience of smoothies. If you do not have the time or are concerned your kids will scoff at the idea of eating whole vegetables and fruits, make smoothies. It is pretty easy to sneak a carrot into a fruit smoothie without destroying the taste of the sweet fruits. Kids love the idea of smoothies and will most likely not even notice the addition of a few vegetables. Maybe a special cup with a straw will encourage your kids to drink their vitamins and minerals. Get creative with your approach: a green smoothie that gives "monster powers" has worked quite well in my family in encouraging picky eaters to get a dose of green leafy vegetables.

It isn't just the simple fact that whole foods are better for you; they have been proven time and again to be very useful in the prevention of numerous illnesses and diseases. Most cancers are considered preventable with a diet rich in fresh fruits and vegetables and whole grains and nuts. Diabetes and heart disease are also preventable with a healthy diet that focuses on eating whole foods rather than foods that are processed and laden with various preservatives that are scientifically proven to be dangerous.

USE OF SYNTHETIC

VITAMINS

It is now highly recommended by health experts to take nutritional supplements that no doubt have numerous benefits. In fact vitamin regimens have been known to treat ailments when taken in proper recommended doses. They are readily available, and the options are endless. As consumers we are being bombarded with advertisements of newer and more effective supplements. Doesn't it feel that you need several supplements to achieve optimal health? The truth is that not all of them are effective or beneficial to you or your children. Have you ever wondered how much money you spend on nutritional supplements for your whole family per year? Should you not spend your hard earned money on things that are good for you? If you have taken some of those synthetic supplements, you probably have noticed that funky neon-colored urine in the bathroom. What is that all about? Should your urine glow in the dark? You already know the answer. Of course it shouldn't! It isn't natural, and this is your body getting rid of products that it does not need. In this case, it is removing the synthetic supplements.

THE PROBLEM

It is common to find that orange juice, cereals, dairy products, and many other foods are fortified with vitamins. The problem with taking certain supplements is not only the dosage but also the quality of the supplements. Extra fortification can lead to toxicity in a healthy individual. It can be as harmful as being deficient. Many of us are unaware of the recommended daily allowance of these vitamins. We assume that if it's fortified with a vitamin, then it must be good. As far as quality is concerned, those that are created in a laboratory (synthetic vitamins) are not completely absorbed by the body and are eliminated, thus causing that neon show in the bathroom. When you think of those capsules sitting in your stomach or in that of your child, waiting to dissolve day after day, it can be very unsettling. Pause for a moment and think about the consequences of constant exposure to something that is not of any benefit to your body and potentially could be harmful.

THE SOLUTION

The absolute best way to get those necessary vitamins and minerals is by eating a proper diet that is rich in whole foods. If you and your family eat a well-rounded diet, there is less pressure to supplement your diet. Look into the Recommended Daily intake (RDI) for vitamins so that you know exactly how much you need and if you prefer to use food alternatives you have to consciously add these foods into your diet. A good resource is The Food and Nutrition Information center. If you have to take supplements, opt for those that are derived from natural sources. If you or your child has a medical condition or are vitamin deficient, please seek medical attention, and take vitamin supplements as prescribed by your physician.

Labels contain many complicated details that are difficult to understand. There are several specific things, however, that will help you navigate the supplement aisle.

1. Some product labels may contain the words "natural," but manufacturers can claim "natural" on their nutritional products

if at least ten percent of the product comes from natural food sources. Check for 100 percent plant or animal-based products.

2. Additionally look for a natural source of these vitamins. Is it from a food source you recognize, such as vitamin A from fish oils or vitamin C from a plant source?

3. Search for words listed in the ingredients that begin with "dl" or end with "ate" or "ide." This indicates it is a synthetic version of the vitamin. Have a look at some of these common synthetic vitamins as they would appear on the ingredient labels.

- **Vitamin A:** acetate and palmitate
- **Vitamin B1 (Thiamine):** thiamine mononitrate, thiamine hydrochloride
- **Pantothenic Acid B5:** calcium d-pantothenate
- **Vitamin B6 (Pyridoxine):** pyridoxine hydrochloride
- **Vitamin C: Ascorbic acid**
- **Choline:** choline chloride, choline bitartrate
- **Vitamin E:** dl-alpha tocopherol, dl-alpha tocopherol acetate or succinate

If you and your family must take supplements, check with a physician, and do your homework to look out for the above warning signs. Do some checking to ensure you are buying supplements from a reputable company. Call the company if you have doubts and ask them if their vitamins are synthetic. Those taking prescription medications need to be aware that supplements can interact with medicines and cause adverse effects. It is also a good idea to stick with one supplement. You don't want five ingredients in one capsule. Avoid buying any supplement that makes outrageous claims. If it sounds too good to be true, it is.

PERSONAL CARE PRODUCTS AND WHY SOME ARE BAD FOR YOU

Personal care products are a necessary part of life, but not all products are created with your health in mind. Companies tend to cater to society's desire to have things as convenient as possible. We are talking about things such as disposable diapers, feminine hygiene products, and other bathroom necessities such as toilet paper.

THE PROBLEM

Babies use diapers for least two years until they are toilet trained. Women, from puberty until menopause, use some form of feminine hygiene product such as pads or tampons. Later in life some may resort to wearing adult diapers for bladder incontinence. These products are convenient, easy to use, and dependable, which is great, except that some of these products come with subtle dangers. Tampons and pads are composed of rayon, cotton, or a combination of both. Rayon is made from bleached wood pulp, the chlorine bleaching of pulp produces a byproduct of the harmful chemical dioxin. Dioxin has been labeled a probable cancer-causing agent. It has a cumulative effect on an individual, permanently affecting their immune system. Dioxins are responsible for a range of reproductive and developmental problems, damaging the immune system, along with causing major hormonal imbalances and cancer. It can be passed to a child through breast milk. Dioxins have also been found in baby diapers. Women and menstruating girls are exposed to this chemical every time they use these products, over twelve thousand tampons or pads will be used over the life time of the average woman.

Toxic shock syndrome has been reported by tampon users even though the numbers of infections have gone down in recent years it still remains a source of concern.

It isn't just the unhealthy aspect of these personal care products we need to consider. Think of the landfills that are loaded with these items. From an environmental perspective, landfills are filled with nonbiodegradable refuse such as diapers and disposable menstrual products wrapped in plastic. There is now a considerable amount of plastic in water bodies as well that are adversely affecting marine life. All you have to do is watch "Animal Planet" to see how human pollution is affecting wildlife and disrupting ecosystems. Landfills are dumped with hundreds of thousands of pounds of human waste seeping into the ground. It is a horrible thought, but it is the cold hard truth. We know human fecal matter, trapped inside diapers that will be around for centuries, contains disease and yet we are filling up our earth with it. You have probably heard that a single disposable diaper takes anywhere from two hundred to five hundred years to break down in a landfill. Nobody knows for sure because they haven't been around that long, but it is safe to say in the forty years or so since disposable diapers have existed, they haven't broken down yet. We may not be suffering today, but generations to come will live to pay for our mistakes. Billions of pads, tampons, and applicators are sent to landfills annually. On an individual level, each of the close to eighty million menstruating people in North America will throw away over twelve thousand disposable pads or tampons in their lifetime. This is a global problem by the way. While organic disposable pads or tampons may be better for your health, they still create the same amount of landfill waste as conventional disposables.

This may sound silly, but have you ever wondered about that smell of diapers fresh out of the box? Most of the time, it is the faint aroma of plastic. We know plastic is toxic. It is a synthetic product made with various chemicals. This is what we are putting on our babies. Some of the side effects of using plastic or disposable diapers include the common rash. The skin of babies is so sensitive. We go to great lengths to protect it. It doesn't make sense that we would wrap them up in fibers and plastics that we know are harmful.

Most of these disposable diapers, even the majority that claim to be biodegradable, contain something called sodium polyacrylate, a type of super absorbent polymer (SAP). This is what holds all the moisture and makes it possible for a baby's skin to remain fairly dry despite urinating several times. You have probably seen this stuff if you have ever experienced a diaper "blowout." Those tiny little crystals or gel beads are what absorb the moisture. Sometimes you may even find these crystals on your baby during a diaper change. For now the safety of this chemical is being debated.

Part of a green lifestyle includes ways of reducing your impact on the environment. Reducing or eliminating the amount of waste you produce is one way you can help lessen the destruction of our earth.

THE SOLUTION

There are solutions that are not only better for the environment and better for your health but also will save you some money!

As I mentioned earlier, it is important to realize that you will not be able to eliminate every potentially harmful chemical from your life, but you may attempt to reduce the exposure to yourself and your loved ones. There is no one-size-fits-all approach because every family is different. Try what works for you.

Cloth diapers are an option and are much safer for your baby's sensitive skin. There are diaper services that take care of all the cleaning for you or you can just do it the way your grandma did. You wash the soiled diapers with detergent that you know is safe for your baby's skin. It isn't difficult, and you will feel much better knowing you are saving money and doing something for the environment. If you go on vacation or are planning a day where you will be out of the house, don't feel bad if you rely on disposable diapers. You are doing what you can and minimally using unbleached, dye-free disposable diapers available at a specialty or health food store. The health of our children is worth the minor inconvenience of washing cloth diapers. An intentionally healthy or green lifestyle should not be a chore that you loathe. If you loathe the work, you will soon abandon it altogether and go back to your old ways. Do what you can and what works best for you!

As women, our feminine health is a big part of our lives. It is something we ought to embrace, accept, and be excited about instead of being burdened. Our monthly cycle is an indication that our body is functioning as it should. Furthermore we need to be aware of the fact that alternative options do exist apart from the widely available disposables. Cloth menstrual pads and a reusable menstrual cup can be used in lieu of the disposable products for your menstrual cycle. Women can look into using cloth panty liners such as Appleliners (www.Appleliners.com) for an alternative to everyday disposable panty liners. In fact these liners work great for everyday use as well as for light incontinence and they come in various styles and colors to suit every woman's life style. These alternatives are economical, reusable, and just as hygienic. These options are environmentally friendly and are safe for you to use without fear of potentially horrible side effects or allergic reactions. Women have been dealing with menstruation for thousands of years without using disposable products. They managed, and so can we. We need to have a positive attitude about how our bodies function and seek products that offer minimal harm. As with all suggestions in this book, be open to exploring, and settle on what works best for you.

TOOTHPASTE

We all want to have clean, sparkling white teeth that are healthy and free of cavities. We have been encouraged to use fluoride among other things to ensure oral health. Commercials advertise toothpaste with whitening capabilities and the benefits of fluoride that is so important to our teeth. Well what is the complete picture? How does all this ultimately affect the overall health of our families?

THE PROBLEM

Fluoride is not entirely safe. It is toxic; it is used in rodenticides and pesticides to kill pests such as rats and insects. In tests on laboratory animals, fluoride has been shown to enhance the brain's absorption of aluminum—the substance that's found in the brains of most Alzheimer's patients. Osteoporosis, musculoskeletal and nervous system ailments, and bone cancer have been linked to excessive fluoridation. Fluoride toothpaste boxes clearly state if your child ingests more than the recommended amount, you need to call the poison control center. Every year, there are more than twenty thousand calls made to the poison control center due to the ingestion of toothpaste. Do you know how much the recommended amount is? You will probably assume the proper amount is a line the length of the bristles. That is what all the commercials show—even the packaging displays. Actually the correct dosage is a pea-sized amount. It is difficult to find commercial toothpaste that doesn't have fluoride in it. Most toothpaste on the shelves today has fluoride in them.

In the United States over seventy percent of the water supply is fluoridated where as in other parts of the world and almost all of Europe they do not fluoridate their water.

Not only is it poisonous when ingested but excess fluoride is also damaging to teeth, causing a condition known as Fluorosis, where teeth become discolored with white spots. Toothpaste marketed to children that is deliciously flavored is especially dangerous. Kids tend to swallow while brushing their teeth. In fact a well-known children's brand toothpaste could kill a child if he ate the entire tube and weighed less than sixty-six pounds. While it is unlikely this scenario would happen, is it a good idea to have toothpaste around that is appealing to children if it could cause them serious harm? A recent article by Dr. Philippe Grandjean, Harvard School of Public Health, and Dr. Philip Landrigan, Icahn School of medicine says that fluoride has been reclassified as a developmental neurotoxin. Children exposed to excess fluoride have shown a reduction in IQ and disruptive behaviors among other things.

THE SOLUTION

Your teeth do not require scrubbing with minty paste riddled with an excess of various harmful chemicals. Celebrities such as Oprah Winfrey have been known to use fluoride-free cleaners such as baking soda. As mentioned earlier, a growing awareness of the risks of fluoride has resulted in healthier options such as fluoride-free toothpaste. A healthy diet and a simple dip of your brush in a bowl of baking soda is more than enough if you wish to stay away from toothpaste that you are unsure about. And what's even better about using plain old baking soda is that it is a natural whitener. If you don't care for the taste, you can add a couple of drops of peppermint essential oil. This is also an antibacterial agent and freshens breath.

You can find fluoride-free toothpaste in a convenient tube readily available in stores. You may have to look for these brands at health food stores. Sea salt and coconut oil are two other options you can use. For children, you can simply brush their little teeth with a dry or wet toothbrush. They don't need toothpaste or baking soda to get their teeth clean.

COSMETICS, PERFUMES, HAIR CARE, AND AEROSOLS

I t is wonderful to want to look and smell good. Good hygiene is something that makes us feel good about ourselves and gives us a boost of self-confidence. However, in our attempt to look and feel a certain way, it would not be wise to do so at the expense of your health. Things like brushing your teeth, washing your skin and hair, and even adding moisture to your skin are all daily activities meant to make you feel and look better. Unfortunately doing these everyday things with certain store-bought products could be hurting your body or even encouraging cancer growth.

Beauty starts on the inside and exudes outward. What we put on our bodies is equally as important as what we put into our bodies. Would you consider eating some of the products you put on your skin? You absolutely should! The skin is the largest organ on our bodies, just as we pay attention to nourish our bodies with healthy food, we should nourish our skin too. It is important to know the potential risk factors associated with the products we use on our bodies so we can make informed decisions. The wonderful thing about knowledge is that it is empowering. Once armed with it, you will be confident about the products you opt for. And most importantly you will know with certainty if an option is good or if it is plain dangerous!

THE PROBLEM

Have you ever wondered how hairsprays or other styling agents make your hair stay set in place? You guessed it: chemicals. These chemicals can seep through your scalp into your bloodstream and throughout your body. Propylene glycol, one of the most common ingredients used in hairstyling products is also used as jet antifreeze in industrial grade. Antifreeze is poisonous. Would you go out to your garage and grab the gallon of antifreeze and spritz it on your hair? No, of course not. It is also used in many other products including food as an additive. It is sad and makes one wonder why hair care product manufacturers are using a chemical that is found in tire sealant, deicers, and adhesives.

I am sure you have experienced holding your breath after using hair spray in your hair. This is your body responding naturally to avoid inhaling the toxic air around you. Before 1970, dangerous carcinogenic ingredients were used in hair products and it took years before they were removed. It has become a common practice in our day for products to be deemed safe and then unsafe after a few years. In the mean time consumers are left as casualties. The chemicals that are currently in use have not been cleared conclusively as the debate continues. At times chemicals are categorized or grouped as fragrance, which in this case does not require listing and therefore makes it extremely difficult to assess their safety. These chemicals can cause eye and lung irritations.

Many of the chemicals used in most of our personal care products are synthetic. These chemicals that make your soap smell good, give it a pretty color, or even make it lather potentially can be dangerous. Ultimately these chemicals can hurt you and your family. These are not abstract ideas; studies have been done in some animals to prove the potentially dangerous side effects of these common chemicals. Numerous scientific studies have been done and are beginning to initiate change. One such change is that the FDA has now banned the use of propylene glycol in or on cat food. Usually when a chemical comes back as something that is potentially harmful, it is tested again and again in an attempt to disprove the nasty side effects. Nonetheless its safety remains questionable. As consumers we have to use extreme caution, which demands that we side with more natural, time-tested alternatives.

What a terrifying nightmare it is for any mom who sends their child to school and gets that dreaded call from the school nurse that your child has head lice. Here begins the search for the right treatment—treatment for the whole family, if I may add that detail. Most of the treatment shampoos on the market have a chemical called lindane. In many parts of the world, this chemical has been banned from the market due to the fact that it can lead to respiratory problems, numbness, seizures, and even death. Lindane is a DDT-related pesticide. Please search DDT-related pesticides online to fully understand the dangers of this product or dangers of lindane itself.

Many of us have become accustomed to having antibacterial soaps and hand sanitizers as staples in our homes, schools, and workplaces. These products have been proven to be no more effective than plain soap and water. In fact more than seventy per-cent of personal care products including liquid soaps, bar soaps, toothpaste, cosmetics, cleansing lotions, acne creams, and wipes contain triclosan or triclocarban. Many health-related disorders have been linked to this chemical after exposure, such as aller-gies, impaired reproduction, hormone disruption, and weakened muscles. There are many chemicals (about eighty thousand!) in many of the products we use that have not been tested fully in the United States for their toxic effects on humans, according to the Natural Resource Defense Council. In April 2013, the *New York Times* ran an article that addressed this issue in depth.

There are, however, some common chemicals that you can look out for on the labels of the products that you buy on a regular basis.

BHA (butylated hydroxyanisole) and BHT (butylated hydroxytoluene) are two chemicals commonly found in food and personal care products. They are preservatives that have been linked to cancer and hyperactivity, especially in children.

P-phenylenediamine is regularly used in hair dyes and dyes in furniture and materials. According to the Center for Disease Control, it is a common allergen that can cause severe breathing problems as well as skin irritations.

DEA (diethanolamine) is often used in shampoos, soaps, lotions, and numerous other cosmetic products. Alone it is fine, but when mixed with other ingredients (for example, in your shampoo) it becomes a carcinogen. It forms a product that is readily absorbed through the skin and has been linked with stomach, esophagus, and liver and bladder cancers.

Dibutyl phthalate is another ingredient regularly used in nail polish. There are links to problems with the male productive system. Pregnant women should avoid using nail polish with this ingredient.

DMDM hydantoin is used in skin creams and tonics, which releases formaldehyde and can cause skin irritation as well as breathing problems.

Diazolidinyl urea is sold as a preservative to keep dangerous pathogens off your skin, but actually releases formaldehyde.

Methenamine is used in eye makeup and is yet another chemical that releases formaldehyde.

Quarternium-15 is used in shampoos and, sadly, even those so-called baby-sensitive bath products. It also releases formaldehyde.

Parabens are regularly found in all cosmetics and shampoos. They are effective at preventing bacteria from growing in the cosmetics, but have been linked to breast cancer. Parabens mimic estrogen, which can result in tumors.

Sodium lauryl sulfate is a regular ingredient in cosmetics, shampoos, and almost every other personal care product. It is known to cause developmental problems, organ toxicity, and there is reason to believe it is a carcinogen when mixed with other chemicals.

Fragrance is a term used to describe chemicals that are used to scent products such as shampoo and deodorant. A single product's secret fragrance mixture can contain potentially hundreds of toxic volatile organic compounds.

Formaldehyde, a known carcinogen, is a common in nail products and in some bath products as well.

Phthalates have been linked to male genital abnormalities, increased rates of childhood asthma, and allergies, including liver and kidney lesions. They are a known hormone disruptor. They are sometimes listed as dibutyl phthalate in nail polish, and can be hidden in the fragrances of many products for adults and children.

Petroleum byproducts are in most personal care products and come in an array of different names. The trepidation is the fact that they are often contaminated by cancer-causing impurities like 1,4-Dioxane. These come as mineral oil, petrolatum, liquid paraffin, toluene, or xylene.

Triclosan is used in antibacterial products and has been linked to the rise of increased bacterial resistance. It also disrupts hormones.

Lead and mercury lead are usually found in makeup such as lipstick and mascara, respectively. They are both neurotoxins.

These are just a handful of chemicals that are used regularly in everything from shampoo to moisturizer to makeup. Each of these ingredients has been linked to some pretty nasty side effects with some that are known to cause cancer. It is heartbreaking to think we are being sold products that could kill us. People work hard for their money, but because of the greed of companies, they are unknowingly hurting themselves and their families by purchasing harmful products. Unfortunately these ingredients are completely legal to use, and companies are not willingly going to create new products without these chemicals if they don't have to. You have to be your own advocate and educate yourself about what is really in that hand cream or that foundation you are spreading on your face.

THE SOLUTION

There are plenty of alternatives to cosmetic products that are supposed to make you beautiful but actually are hurting you. One of the easiest solutions to the need for hairspray is to try a more natural style. Fortunately, there are plenty of hairstyles that are currently "in" that require little to no hair products to achieve the look. Many new brands are offering much safer products without the harmful chemicals. If you really need some kind of hold for your hair, try flaxseed. When boiled with water, flaxseed creates a hair gel that offers great hold. Or try one hundred percent pure aloe vera gel. If your goal is to hold your curls throughout the day, you can mix one to four teaspoons of sea salt and about one cup of water in a small spray bottle. These methods are safe, natural, and effective.

As far as cosmetics go, there are plenty of ways to add a little color to your face without hurting yourself with harsh chemicals. You can purchase make up free of the above listed ingredients online or in stores. How many times do you see a cosmetic product highlighting an ingredient when in reality it is the fifth or second to last ingredient on the label? It is very simple to make your own skincare products with a few ingredients you probably already have in your kitchen. Olive oil, coconut oil, grape seed oil and honey are great for your skin. If you would like something less greasy add aloe vera gel to the mix and blend together into a fluffy airy lotion. It is easy and a great way to avoid fillers and harmful chemicals like mineral oil which is a byproduct of petroleum and is harmful to the skin. If you like scented lotions, you can add a little essential oil such as lavender for something extra. If you are not one of those DIY people, many small companies and newer brands are offering good quality products to make this jump easy for you.

DANGERS OF PERFUME

Perfume is meant to make you smell better, which often gives you a little extra self-confidence and lifts your spirits. But smelling good shouldn't hurt you, and unfortunately some perfumes are made with ingredients that are harmful to your skin. For example ninety five percent of chemicals used in fragrances are synthetic compounds derived from petroleum. These chemicals include benzene derivatives, aldehydes, and many other known toxins and sensitizers capable of causing cancer, birth defects, central nervous system disorders, and allergic reactions.

The most obvious side effect of some of the most popular commercial fragrances is a rash. Some people are allergic to the strong scents that are in most perfumes. Asthma attacks or sneezing fits are common for the perfume wearer as well as those around them.

Here are some basic facts that you may not know about your favorite perfume. In the perfume industry, there are about five thousand different chemicals used to make those precious scents. Of those five thousand, only about 20 percent have been tested to see if they are safe for humans to wear on their skin or breathe in. Some of the chemicals are known toxins. You might be thinking that every perfume we wear must be safe. The only ones responsible for making sure the perfume is safe are the ones who make the perfumes, and they are not required by the Food and Drug Administration to test for safety. It doesn't exactly make you feel very safe does it?

Before you run and check the label to see if there are ingredients in your perfume that are harmful, I have to tell you something else. You are not going to like it. Fragrances rarely include a complete, comprehensive list of every chemical that is used to make it. One study found that, on average, there are fourteen chemicals left off the label. These chemicals can be linked to allergic reactions as well as hormone disruption. As we all know hormones help our bodies function normally and are necessary in reproduction among other functions. When there is a malfunction in this process things start to go awry. Women experiencing hormonal imbalances or menopause know this all too well and attempt to correct their hormone function. Headaches and nausea are common side effects of inhaling certain perfumes. This is essentially an allergic reaction. Your body is telling you it doesn't like the chemical reaction that is happening and is giving you the signals to avoid it in the future.

THE SOLUTION

Just because some perfumes are dangerous doesn't mean you can't still smell good. You can make your own fragrance, tailored to your tastes and your personality. Isn't that what a signature scent is all about? Do you like floral scents that are more traditional and romantic or maybe something fruity and fun? This can be achieved by mixing your own special scent in your kitchen. Make a variety of different fragrances to suit your mood or seasons.

All you need is a carrier oil such as jojoba or almond oil to which you will add an essential oil. Use a bottle with a dark tint because dark bottles will preserve perfume longer and keep light from weakening it.

These oils are safe to use on your skin in carrier oil and are much better than alcohol, which is the typical base of commercial perfumes. Take a moment to browse the essential oil section in your local organic store or online. Pick a couple of scents that you like and that will complement each other. When creating a fragrance, always remember to do a skin patch test especially if you are new to a particular essential oil. Pregnant women are to be cautious as certain essential oils can cause stimulation of the bladder and uterus, always read the label. The rule of thumb is to choose a base note, middle note, and top note scent. The base is the scent that will hold the longest on your skin. The middle note, not surprisingly, is what you smell between the top and base notes. The top note is the scent you get when you first spritz the perfume on. It will evaporate fairly quickly.

Do some experimenting, and have fun with it. It is exciting to make a scent that suits your personal tastes. Your friends will wonder what you are wearing, and you will be able to tell them that it is your own special blend. Don't be surprised if they ask you to make them some. And the best thing about it is that it is all natural. Many companies online do offer readymade healthy eco-friendly perfumes.

CHOOSING SAFE
FURNITURE

Furniture is not technically a necessity in life, but it certainly makes life easier. It is nice to sit around a table and enjoy a family dinner or relax on the sofa with a good book. However, just as we need to make knowledgeable decisions about our food or personal care products, we ought to know that even furniture purchasing has to be based not just on the price, aesthetic quality, or features but also on what raw materials were used as well as the treatment it underwent. Not all furniture is safe. Wood, leather, and various other fabrics are sometimes treated with chemicals during the manufacturing process. These resins and other chemicals are toxic and although you may not be consuming them, when they are sitting in your home, vapors are released into the air. You can't see them, and you probably can't smell them especially over time, but they certainly are there.

THE PROBLEM

Most furniture is treated with fire-retardant chemicals to meet established fire safety standards. Unfortunately if there ever is a fire and that furniture is burned, it releases more harmful chemicals into the air. According to studies, many flame-retardant chemicals raise health concerns, including cancer, hormone disruption, and harmful effects on brain development. Furniture treated with these flame-retardant chemicals are sitting in our living rooms and poisoning our children and us.

It is a proven fact that the chemicals that are released into the air during the manufacturing, use, and disposal of furniture cause some serious health problems. It is said that women may have a harder time conceiving due to chemical exposure. Babies may be born with lower IQs or develop Attention Deficit Disorder. Serious illnesses in children have been linked to these chemicals. Male infertility is another common side effect of the chemicals used to make our furniture "safer." You would expect dust or mold to trigger an allergic response, but few people expect their furniture, carpet, or kitchen cabinets to cause an asthma attack.

In some cases, the furniture you buy is safe. Once you have it home, however, maintaining the couch with cleaners ends up making the couch unsafe. Chemicals in the cleaner are absorbed by the fabric, and the vapors are inhaled as you lay your face on the couch or as your little one curls up on the sofa with his favorite blanket right on the spot where the chemicals have been poured.

Your bookshelves, entertainment stands, and even your dressers may be furniture loaded with harsh chemicals. Formaldehyde is used regularly to treat particleboard. Formaldehyde can bring on an asthma attack in those who are prone to breathing problems. Particleboard is an inexpensive material commonly used for furniture. These are the items you would pick up at most regular stores. Some of the more expensive wood products are often made with real wood but may contain their own problems due to the stains used on the wood.

Composite board and plywood are also treated with formaldehyde. This chemical substance is a favorite among manufacturers because it has strong adhesive and preservative properties. Some hardwood flooring may also contain this toxic substance.

Curtains are another item that tends to be treated with flame-retardant chemicals. All of these treatments are meant to keep us safe, but they are only harming us in the long run. PVC (polyvinyl chloride) window blinds, especially those that are manufactured in certain foreign countries, tend to include lead and carcinogens. Stick with blinds that are made in the United States or Canada. They typically do not contain lead.

THE SOLUTION

I hope you are not feeling like there is just no way out of this complicated mess. You don't have to resort to sitting on the floor or throwing out your sofa today. However you can take some precautions to try and lessen the effect of those chemicals. Air out your home as much as you can, especially after purchasing new furniture. This allows fresh air to sweep through your home.

Many offending chemicals off-gas at higher rates when humidity and temperature are higher. Keep the humidity below 45 percent. Avoid eating while sitting on your couch. Use a vacuum with a HEPA (high-efficiency particulate absorption) filter on the carpets and furniture to try to get out some of the dangerous lint. Whenever possible, use a damp cloth to wipe down your furniture to remove some of the toxins that build up. If you are in a position to buy new furniture, do a little research first. Look into furniture that is made with green materials. When you head to the furniture store, read the labels on the furniture. California has a unique flammability standard, TB 117. Look for any signs or labels on furniture that indicate TB 117 has been used to treat the furniture. This is the flame-retardant chemical that is sprayed on the foam and stuffing in the furniture. Unfortunately, there are still some companies that use TB 117 but don't indicate it on the label. One of the best ways to ensure your sofa is not treated with TB 117 is to buy vintage. By *vintage*, I mean it was made before 1975. Of course, it is difficult to find furniture that old, but if grandma's couch is still around, it wouldn't hurt to reupholster and use it. Look for furniture that has not been treated with harmful chemicals. There are many options out there.

For your shelving needs, look for products that are made with natural wood. Avoid any furniture made of pressboard or MDF (medium density fiberboard). MDF contains urea-formaldehyde, which is a probable carcinogen and may cause allergies, especially if one inhales the dust. If newer products are more expensive, you may want to look into buying secondhand furniture. Scour yard sales, thrift stores, and other recycling centers. Things have become significantly easier due to more companies opting to avoid these "sticky" chemicals. It is important not to assume that something is safe but to confirm before you make a purchase.

CLOTHING AND TOXINS

When you look good, you feel good. When your children look nice, you feel a sense of pride. On special occasions, we dress our little ones up so they will look picture perfect. Often we will go out and splurge a bit to buy a new dress or suit so they will look extra special. When we are browsing through the mall, it is hard to resist new outfits because they are just too cute! Buying clothes for you and your family is necessary, but I hope from now on what you buy is something you will carefully consider; not all clothes are created equal.

THE PROBLEM

Most of us don't even think twice about our clothing hurting us. As moms, we often rub a piece of clothing on our face to test the softness and determine whether or not it is too abrasive for our kid's sensitive skin. But did you know some clothing is actually made with toxic chemicals? These chemicals are absorbed through the skin and into your blood system where serious damage then happens.

Last year a study was done that included the testing of 141 different garments manufactured in twenty-nine different countries. Of the garments tested, eighty-nine tested positive for nonylphenol ethoxylates, or NPEs. These chemicals are hormone disruptors. As you have read through this book, you have probably noticed some of the biggest chemical offenders are hormone disruptors. This is very serious and can lead to all kinds of developmental problems as well as certain cancers.

A small percentage of the clothing tested was positive for carcinogens and phthalates. The clothing tested wasn't just cheap stuff you would expect to be manufactured in a third-world country. No, these are brands you know and probably love, including high-end designers. Knowledge is power. I strongly encourage you to read and to do more research into NPEs.

You probably already know about the flame-retardant chemicals that are used on almost all clothing. These may be listed on the tag as PBDEs, or antimony polybrominated diphenyl ethers. Along with various skin irritations such as hives and rashes, the chemicals are known to cause birth defects and fertility issues. In fact, the chemicals that are supposed to save us in a fire are hurting us in our daily lives. There is an entire laundry list of side effects that are associated with PBDEs. Fleece, cotton, and polyester regularly are treated with flame-retardant chemicals.

Dry cleaners have been known to use a chemical called perchlorethylene which has been linked to cancer, liver and kidney damage. The Environmental Protection agency EPA, has determined that it is a "likely" carcinogen. Consider constant and prolonged exposure to clothes cleaned in this product.

Along with the above common chemicals in clothes, there are plenty more that you would never know about unless you did some research.

* Fluoride ends up on your clothing after you wash it in water treated with the chemical.

*Heavy metals are often used in dyes. These metals include lead, nickel, and chrome.

*Dyes often contain carcinogens.

*Fungicides are known toxins. You are advised to wear gloves and coveralls when dealing with fungicides.

* Formaldehyde is used as an antiwrinkle agent. The chemical is extremely harmful to the brain.

* Antibacterial chemicals are often used in sportswear. They are supposed to keep the garments from smelling during heavy sports play. Unfortunately the chemicals cause rashes, and their production is harmful to aquatic life.

THE SOLUTION

While it is nice to think you could buy completely organic clothing for your family, that is often not feasible. Organic materials are those that have not been treated with harsh chemicals. There are quite a few manufacturers who use organic cotton and hemp. Some wool is also toxin free. The organic cottons are colored with low-impact dyes, which are better for your skin and the environment.

If you do buy clothing off the rack, it is always a good idea to wash it at least once before you or your family members wear it. Flame-retardant chemicals and other toxins, however, can take more than fifty washes before all traces are gone. It is also a good idea to buy vintage or used clothing. Remember to use a good detergent to wash your clothes—one that does not contain harmful chemicals in them. Do find out from your dry cleaner if they use eco-friendly and healthy products on your clothes. Avoid dry cleaners that do not mention that they adhere to safe, environmentally friendly practices.

LAUNDRY PRODUCTS

Laundry, laundry, laundry! Oh how I can't stand to do our laundry at times, but I have to. How dirty do your clothes truly get on a daily basis? Maybe your kids were rolling in the mud, or you were working out at the gym. You probably feel like you need something really strong to do the job. Luckily—or unluckily—for us consumers, there is something for everyone on the market depending on our needs. Manufacturers offer to sell us laundry detergent that is meant to be tough on dirt. If it is tough on dirt, guess what else it is tough on? Your skin and the skin of your family is being given the same treatment as those nasty stains. Do you really want to have your little ones wearing something that can actually cause them pain or discomfort in future? Of course you don't.

THE PROBLEM

Laundry soap is one of the harshest products in our homes. Many are made with known harmful ingredients including dyes and fragrances. Manufacturers are not required by law to disclose the list of ingredients used. Fabric softener and bleach are also harsh to our skin. It makes no sense that we would want those harsh chemicals rubbing against our skin day in and day out. Did you know that some of the chemical ingredients in some common household name-brand detergents are actually known to cause cancer? If you didn't know before, you know now. Findings by University of Washington researchers published online in the journal Air Quality, Atmosphere and Health report that air vented from machines using scented laundry detergents and dryer sheets release gases containing acetaldehyde and benzene which are classified by the Environmental Protection Agency EPA as carcinogens.. Wouldn't you like to find another way to clean your clothes without fear of triggering allergies or skin reactions or even cancer?

THE SOLUTION

It is only natural you would want your clothing to look as good as it did the day you bought it. Excessive washing and washing with harsh cleaners, however, destroy the fabric over time. You can prolong the life of your clothing by reverting to a practice our grandparents and their parents used. Have specific wardrobes for the various activities in your life.

Clothes that are stained are not necessarily ruined. Set these clothes aside for cleaning around the house or for the kids to play in. Save your good, unsullied clothing for school, work, or running errands. Have a few versatile pieces for your church wardrobe or special evenings out. This is an excellent way to preserve your clothing, and you will not need to use harsh cleansers to try and get rid of every stain, especially on designated play clothes.

Another incentive for finding alternatives to soaps like the regular ones that you have probably been using is the money you can save by choosing safer options. It is so incredibly easy to make your own laundry soap with just a couple of ingredients, but you also can purchase readily available healthier detergent options. I love ECOS laundry detergent, it is clearly labeled and comes with built in fabric softener. Soap nuts are another great option. These nuts grow on trees and have been used in Asia and are easily available for purchase online or in certain stores. Simply ask the store attendants for help in the laundry aisle. They come in a bag that you toss into your laundry. They are extremely economical and can be reused several times before simply discarding the biodegradable nuts. Eco balls or wash balls are another way of reducing chemical exposure as well as saving money and energy while you do your laundry. These balls are designed in such a way that you simply harness the cleaning power of water without the use of any kind of detergent. The balls use an ionization cleaning process that is a result of the motion of the washing machine agitator and the water. They can be found in the laundry aisle and last up to sixty loads of laundry. According to the company's website they claim they will last up to a thousand washes.

Dryer balls save you from chemical exposure and help dry your clothes efficiently in the dryer without using fabric softener or dryer sheets. As with any change, know what is realistic for you, and make changes accordingly.

CLEANING THE HOUSE

Your home is your castle and your sanctuary. We take great pride in having a comfortable, clean, and most importantly, safe home for our families. Cleanliness is important to our overall health. We know this, and many of us attempt to maintain a somewhat regular cleaning routine and schedule. If you walk down the supermarket aisles, you will discover the endless offerings of cleaning products. The options are overwhelming, but upon further inspection, you will realize many are very similar in their ingredient compositions. Many years ago I would choose the most potent cleansers at the supermarket without any consideration of their toxicity. If I needed an oven cleaner, I needed one that would do the job fairly quickly and sufficiently. I only read to find out details about what it could do. Yes, I coughed through the fumes, but I was more concerned about making sure my oven was spotlessly clean. The question I never asked myself was whether or not the bleach and the fumes in these cleaning products could hurt us. As a society, we have become extremely obsessed with cleaning our homes with toxic chemicals that are intended to keep us healthy by eliminating germs. These cleaning products kill not only the bad bacteria but also the good bacteria and subtly poison our bodies. Our primary concern should not be to provide a sterile environment but instead to provide a safe one that promotes good health.

THE PROBLEM

This is the part those brilliant labels on the carpet cleaners don't tell you. Every time you clean your carpet with one of those intense cleaners in an attempt to remove all the bacteria, dirt, and grime on your floor, you are leaving behind something so much more dangerous: toxic waste. The chemicals in the cleaners are left behind and are absorbed into the padding under your carpet as well as the carpet fibers. When you walk on your carpet, you are coming into contact with the chemicals. Your little ones are playing on a toxic minefield. Imagine having a great time tickling your children as you all roll on the floor with giggles. Sadly, you are rolling on toxins that can hurt your lungs, damage the brain, and can even cause cancer. It certainly ruins the fun of the moment when you think about it like that.

Think about the smell of these cleaning products. Sometimes the vapors are so strong that they make your eyes water and your nostrils burn. You might notice you suddenly develop a dry cough. This is not a good thing! Why would we want to cause ourselves pain and suffering to clean our homes? Is it OK that we have to ventilate the bathroom when we are using some powerful cleaning agent on the toilet? No! It is certainly not OK, and it should set off a string of warning bells. If it is doing that to you, imagine your children's little bodies and what those vapors are doing to it. We know vapors go straight to the brain. Chemicals that are certainly not good for your neurological health are bombarding your brain. Think of the headache you get when you are scrubbing the tiles in your bathroom. That is your brain screaming at you to get clean air because toxic chemicals are overwhelming it. At times the cleaning products may be sweetly scented like a lemon, which may make you feel good but doesn't take away from the harsh reality. It is important to read the ingredient labels to check for the bad chemicals but also the instructions, which are a good indicator as to whether you should be using certain cleaners. In most cases the presence of the bad disqualifies the good. Most of the time, the good ingredients will be highlighted, whereas the truth of the matter is that it may only constitute a minimal percentage of the product. Aerosols, for example, can be fatal if inhaled. Most cans will say not to use in a small, unventilated area. That is a red flag right there.

Creating a sterile environment creates a slew of health problems as you destroy even those microorganisms that are of benefit to your health.

If you research the ingredients in your cleaning products, you will be floored at how toxic they are. The Environmental Working Group has a list on their website about some of the worst cleaners. Check out www.ewg.org.

These cleaners are known to contain carcinogens. Sparkling clean toilets may be contributing to the incidences of cancer.

*Some toilet bowl cleaners are packed with chlorine. You are supposed to use gloves to handle them. They are toxic and fatal if swallowed. Others are acidic and can cause "irreversible damage" if a drop gets in your eye during cleaning.

*Some laundry detergents contain formaldehyde. These laundry detergents may be inexpensive, but they are not worth the risk.

*Some tarnish removers are downright lethal and have been declared carcinogens. Try using salt, baking soda, and hot water to clean your silver.

*Some jewel cleaners are toxic and are believed to be carcinogens. Imagine putting your necklace or ring on after it has been soaking in a cancer-causing solution.

*Some multisurface and floor cleaners are very dangerous; they are banned for use in most countries, but not the United States. Chemicals in the cleaner break down into something known as nonylphenol, which interferes with the hormonal system.

*A common bathroom cleanser is banned in Europe, but sold every day in the United States. The chemicals in the cleaner irritate and inflame the lungs.

*Some floor cleaners contain fifteen times the allowable amount of methoxydiglycol that is allowed in Europe. It is linked to harming fetuses. It is still on store shelves in the United States.

*A common mildew stain remover plus blocker is not sold in Canada or Europe because it contains 2-butoxyethanol which is suspected to be carcinogenic.

*Certain fume-free oven cleaners are not quite as safe as the label would have you believe. It can and will hurt your lungs. If you have used any oven cleaner, you know how horrible this stuff smells and how it hurts your skin and lungs.

Those are just a handful of products. These made the list because they are the worst. **That does not mean the other cleaners are safe**; they just happen to be less deadly. Any product that comes with a warning of danger should be avoided. Some may indicate that even the vapors are harmful. All of these labels should be taken seriously. You don't need that stuff in your home.

THE SOLUTION

It is possible to clean your home with a little soap and water without hurting you or your family? Whenever I walk through the cleaning aisle in search of my favorite castile soap, I am amazed by the constantly evolving labels on the products. It is rather intimidating as you see the claims boasted by each product and the sheer number of products used for different areas of the home. There are cleaners for your kitchen sink, the kitchen floor, the toilet, the bathtub, the carpet, and on and on. It is a mind-boggling experience.

Do you know how many cleaning products you really need to have in your home? You can thoroughly and beautifully clean your home with only three products: castile soap, Vinegar, and baking soda.Water happens to be the star of this show by the way. You also can add lemon juice to the list of cleaning supplies, if you'd like. Castile soap works as a multipurpose cleaner for the home and its gentle enough to use on your body. One part Vinegar to one part water in a spray bottle with a citrus essential oil makes a great disinfectant, degreaser and deodorizer. Your oven will be thoroughly cleaned with baking soda left to work over a few hours. Think about how much space you need in your home to devote to storing your cleaning products. You also have to store the chemical cleaners somewhere the kids can't get into because they are poisonous. Imagine the space you can free up by getting rid of the myriad of products. And imagine relieving the stress of worrying about what will happen if your little one manages to get his or her hands on your kitchen cleaner. It is exciting to realize how much money you will save by not buying all those cleaning products several times a year.

If you are not willing to do the completely natural cleaning method, there are some products you can buy that are much safer than the standard chemical-laden cleaner. Don't worry about not jumping in totally to the green thing. Baby steps will work. When looking for "green" cleaners, read the labels carefully as well as the ingredients. Choose products that use plant-based ingredients. Stay away from ammonia or chlorine in the ingredient list.

Do not buy into a beautifully packaged product that touts things like "green" or "eco-friendly." Look for specifics. You want the product to specify there are no solvents or phosphates. Phosphates are very harmful to the environment. If it includes the term *biodegradable*, it should say how long it takes for the product to break down. It is easy to label anything biodegradable because everything breaks down eventually, but will it happen in one year or five hundred years?

PREGNANCY

Pregnancy is an exciting time in a woman's life. It is usually a time of anticipation, exploration, and much preparation. An expecting mother has so much to think about during those nine months. Thoughts of excitement for her growing baby, what adjustments she will need to make in her life, her health and that of the baby are some of the many thoughts that cross her mind as she prepares to bring a new life into the world. She is dealing with her body morphing and a deep sense of responsibility to prepare for her baby.

Pregnant mothers are encouraged to avoid certain foods and drinks that are known to be detrimental to the development of the fetus. Bad habits such as smoking and drinking are also strongly discouraged. Moms-to-be are asked to hold off on beauty routines such as hair coloring. This precaution is to give the unborn child the best chance of being born healthy. There are two facts about life that are true: there are things we can control, and there are things we can't control. It is wise to focus on those things that we can control, one of them being the environment you create for this new baby. What a privilege and an opportunity to ensure that your baby has a good start in a safe environment that promotes good health.

THE PROBLEM

It is nearly impossible to get away from every single carcinogen in the environment, but it is imperative to understand that an unborn baby can be exposed to harmful chemicals even while in the uterus. Every unborn baby has a chance to be healthy by avoiding some of the most common chemical offenders, such as biphenyl A (BPA), which has been in the news recently. Many ideas are being tossed around regarding how to avoid its use in the production of certain products such as the cans our canned food is stored in or plastic food storage containers.

Our lack of awareness does not minimize the exposure to harmful chemicals. For example, in our quest to save food in our refrigerators, how many of us have used storage containers such as Tupperware? According to Tupperware, only their products sold after March 2010 are free of BPA. I am sure none of us ever considered these food containers as a source of potential danger to our health and that of our loved ones. BPA causes problems for the human brain and prostate. It also has been linked to cancer, diabetes, obesity, reproductive problems, and early onset of puberty. It has been "considered safe in low doses," though in reality it still remains questionable. I wonder if any moms are willing to put their trust in a manufacturer's unverifiable claim that only the minimum amount of BPA was used in a given product. It is a risky game that is best avoided altogether. The Center for Disease Control confirms that more than ninety percent of the American population has measurable amounts of BPA in their system. A study reported by the *Journal of the American Medical Association* (JAMA) reported in 2008 that exposure to BPA was linked to an increase in cardiovascular diseases, type 2 diabetes, and liver enzyme abnormalities. And these effects were seen at relatively low-dose amounts of BPA—well below the amount consumed by Americans on a daily basis. There are plenty of products on the market that are free of BPA and are comparable in cost to those that contain the harmful chemical. Once again, you have to be aware and conscious about this fact when purchasing plastic products.

Another chemical pregnant women need to be cautious of is lead. It may be in paint or the pipes in your home, especially if it is a building built prior to 1978. Another place you may not expect to find lead is your garden hose. In fact many hoses contain a label that reveals there may be lead present. This opens up a whole new set of problems. You water your garden with the hose, you fill up the kiddie pool, and you may even snag a quick drink of water from the hose. Please don't do this. There are hoses on the market that do not contain lead. They are a few dollars more, but well worth the cost.

Lead pipes leech lead into your tap water. Ingesting lead during pregnancy can cause a miscarriage, low birth weight, or premature birth. Lead may be present in antique dishes and ceramics. Scented candles also may be harmful to your unborn baby because the wicks may contain lead. Although it is natural for many moms to get into nesting mode, they may want to undertake home renovations before the baby comes. You may want to consider the products being used, especially the organic solvents commonly found in degreasers, paint thinners, and varnish removers. These include alcohols, toluene, benzene, xylene, and ethers, which are all potentially dangerous to the baby.

Some chemicals, such as diethyltoluamide (DEET), are absorbed into your skin. DEET is a pesticide commonly used in mosquito repellents. If you must use DEET spray, spray your clothing instead of your skin, or opt for products free of these chemicals.

Mercury is another concerning heavy metal. Mercury is a known neurotoxin. Fish usually ingest mercury. Most doctors advise pregnant women to avoid eating certain kinds of fish: shark, king mackerel, swordfish, and tilefish. It is not wise for pregnant women or those planning on becoming pregnant to entirely avoid all kinds of fish from their diet. Fish contains many healthy nutrients that are essential for growth and development, especially in a pregnant mom and baby.

Another offender comes in the form of cookware. Teflon chemicals that are emitted by nonstick cookware can cause cancer, obesity, and low birth weight.

Arsenic poisoning is more common than you would think or want to believe. Even though it is readily found in nature, overexposure during pregnancy can cause miscarriage, birth defects, or stillbirths. Your gorgeous backyard complete with wooden swing sets for the kids and those picnic tables may be riddled with arsenic. Arsenic was used routinely as a preservative in pressure-treated lumber used for building decks and play structures. Even your wood deck may be harboring this deadly chemical. Wood is often treated with arsenic-containing stains. We talked about being cautious with wood a little earlier in the furniture section. If you live in a rural farming area, the risk of being exposed to arsenic in fertilizer is quite high. If you have a private well, make sure you have it tested regularly to ensure arsenic has not leaked into your water supply. This happens more often than you may realize.

Chlorinated tap water has been linked to a lot of health conditions such as asthma, eczema and various cancers such as breast, colon and rectal among several others. According to the U.S Council of Environmental Quality "cancer risks among people drinking chlorinated water is ninety three percent higher than among those whose water does not contain chlorine." Unfortunately it can be absorbed through your skin while taking a shower or drinking tap water.

THE SOLUTION

The previous section may be a little terrifying, but you can limit your exposure to these toxins by changing your habits and simply by being more aware of your surroundings. You can avoid the majority of these chemicals by being proactive; watch what you eat and what you use to cook and store your food in. Cast-iron cookware is great cookware because it adds iron to your meals, which can help prevent anemia. Have your pipes inspected by a plumber if you suspect they may be lead especially if you live in an older home built before 1950. Additionally have your water tested to search for chemicals mentioned above, whether you have a well or use city water. Although it may not be feasible for you to move or to have your pipes redone in your home, you can use a water filter to limit the amount of chemicals you ingest. A water filter for your drinking water as well as one for your shower will help do the job.

Avoid using plastic reusable containers that contain BPA. Look at the bottom of any plastic container. If there is a number three or seven on it, don't use it. Only use numbers four, five, one and two for food items. It is also a good idea to avoid using plastics to reheat food in a microwave. There are toxins in the plastic that are released when the plastic is heated. If you have the means, build a deck made out of natural wood that hasn't been treated with a treatment that contains arsenic. If your deck is treated, try to make it impossible for children to get under the deck. These are inviting play spots for little ones, but the arsenic from the wood treatment can leech into the soil below the deck. Have your husband or somebody who is not pregnant seal the wood every six months. This will help prevent the arsenic from escaping onto your skin or food. Throw a tablecloth over your picnic table, and make sure you wash your hands really well after touching the wood. This will help reduce your exposure to the arsenic. Never allow your food to come in direct contact with the wood

If you must do projects around the home opt for healthy and eco-friendly supplies. Ask the store attendant at your hardware store to help you with these selections. Knowledge is power, and once you know the risk, you can take steps to minimize it. Pay close attention to labels, and avoid buying products that may contain lead. Be wary of old costume jewelry as well. It may have been your great grandmother's, but there is a strong possibility it may contain lead. Most of the newer jewelry on the market today does not contain lead, however, there are still a few manufacturers that continue to use lead. Be aware of what chemicals may be around you; a small amount of vigilance will greatly benefit your health.

KIDS' EXPOSURE TO TOXINS IN TOYS AND PLASTIC BOTTLES

We have all experienced little children putting everything into their mouth—and I mean *everything*. Although a toy may look clean, its safety is a whole other thing. Not all toys are created equal; just because they are being sold in a store does not mean they are always safe. Toys are painted to be bright and colorful, which is very attractive for babies and toddlers. We teach them colors using these toys, they see, they touch, and sometimes it goes right into the mouth. We want our children to enjoy their childhood and enjoy the many fun toys available on the market. It is exciting to give your little one a new toy that you know will keep him busy for hours. However, toys can get quite expensive, and at times we may look for cheaper alternatives. This is not to say that expensive toys are the best toys, but this is where things may start to get dicey.

TOYS

Toys managed to go unregulated for years for some reason or other. Thank God there are more guidelines now than there were in the past regarding toy safety. No one can protect your children like you can. The responsibility is on the parents to ensure that their children are playing with toys that are safe and stimulate their little brains. We have had labels warning of choking hazards for years, but that is only half the problem. Too many toys have been put out on the market only to be recalled later for containing toxins or other defect that could harm a child. Sadly at times it has taken accidents and deaths for recalls to occur. That is a price parents should not have to pay.

THE PROBLEM

Unfortunately, the plastics baby toys are made with combined with the paint that gives the toys those bright colors is not always safe. In fact some of the bottles we use to feed our little ones often are made with chemicals that are dangerous and known to cause various health problems. Sadly toys are being put onto the market with chemicals such as cadmium and lead present. We have talked about the dangers of lead and how harmful it is, and while there are guidelines imposed, manufacturers get around these by having their toys made in foreign countries where the guidelines are very lax.

Most girls go through a stage where they like to play dress up. They adorn themselves in cute little outfits and jewelry. They are beautiful and it is fun to see them dressed up. Unfortunately, a lot of the pretend jewelry that is made for kids is made with lead. It isn't just costume jewelry made for kids; that inexpensive kitschy stuff at mall stores is often made with lead. Little pieces are easy to swallow and can wreak havoc on a little one's system. In one situation, a six-year-old died after swallowing a tiny heart-shaped lead charm and developing lead poisoning. These are terrible stories, and nobody wants to hear them, but we must. We must learn from these tragic deaths and realize the problem is very real. The child doesn't even need to swallow the lead to be harmed by it. Sucking on toys or jewelry that are coated with paint that contains lead can cause developmental delays and flu-like symptoms.

Cobalt, like many trace elements, is useful to the body in trace amounts. It is an element used in many blue dyes and has been found in some building blocks and bibs. The problem occurs when there is overexposure to cobalt. Overexposure to cobalt can lead to asthma and several respiratory irritations among other conditions. In one study, it was found in the urine of some babies.

Phthalates are another substance that is banned for use in toys, but are still there. They are a combination of man-made chemicals commonly found in plastic toys manufactured before 2008. Considering most toys are plastic, this is quite scary. Phthalates have been linked to some developmental disorders, chronic asthma, and diabetes. Although this nasty stuff has been banned from toys, phthalates are still used in binders, lunch boxes, backpacks, and other school supplies, which is baffling because young children are getting exposed.

THE SOLUTION

You obviously don't want your child to be licking toys coated with lead. Do your homework and read the packaging of any toy before you buy it. A few good toys that cost a little more but are completely safe for your child are always going to be better than many toys that are inexpensive and deadly. Fortunately our government has realized lead poisoning is a serious matter, and there are some regulations in place to help limit the amount of lead in toys. Keep in mind, though, that this applies to the United States, and not all companies manufacture their goods here.

And there are plenty of manufacturers who are breaking these regulations and putting lead in the toys anyway. One report you can check regularly is the Trouble in Toyland list or check www.watoxics.org for further reading. Toys that are new and popular may be dangerous. Check the list first before you buy and share the list with family and friends. Many of the regulations are fairly new, so toys from your oldest child may not have been safe and are not OK to use for your new baby or to give away.

When buying plastic toys, lunch boxes, or anything else for your child, avoid buying anything that has the number three in the center of the triangle. Numbers one, two, four, and five are deemed safe. If you have toys that have been around for more than four years, it is strongly recommended you avoid giving them to children. It is just too hard to verify that they are safe before giving them to your little one.

Another option is to give your children toys that are made with safe, natural sources. Untreated wood blocks, cars, and puzzles are excellent options. Dolls made with organic material are ideal. If you can name it, you can probably find it manufactured in a way that will not hurt your child. Look for companies that sell green, organic, or nontoxic toys. You will feel much better knowing your little one isn't chewing on something that could hurt his or her development.

BOTTLES

Bottles are a necessity. The choices are endless, which is great! We must have them to feed our little ones. We go to great lengths to sterilize them and clean them between uses. All of this is in order to keep the wee ones from getting sick. Unfortunately the bottle itself can make the baby sick, and each time you heat the plastic bottle for sterilization, you may be making the problem worse.

THE PROBLEM

The problem is the plastic, or what is used to make the plastic: that nasty thing we mentioned earlier known as BPA which a 2010 report from the U.S Food and drug Administration (FDA) identified as a possible hazard to fetuses, infants and young children. Typically babies want warm milk. When you heat the bottles to warm the milk, BPA is released, and the baby ingests it while they are enjoying their dinner. Despite the government recognizing the dangers of BPA, it has still not been banned and is used regularly in products. It wasn't until 2012 that a ban on BPA in baby bottles was instated. Bottles manufactured before the ban, however, are still available.

And, unfortunately, it isn't just BPA that raised concerns in those plastic bottles but also phthalates which have been known to produce adverse effects on the reproductive system. Plastic is a man-made product, which means chemicals are always going to be present. One study said that now that manufacturers are being forced to eliminate BPA, they are substituting it with chemicals that have not been tested fully. The study proved that ninety five percent of plastic found in bottles, sippy cups, and a variety of other products all contained chemicals that produced a pseudo-estrogen. Synthetic hormones are dangerous. These are released when there is a change of temperature, such as exposure to sunlight or dishwashing.

THE SOLUTION

While it would be easy to suggest tossing out all of your plastic bottles, I know that is pretty tough to do. Glass bottles are a great option, but you may think they are an accident waiting to happen once the baby starts to hold his own bottle. However, glass bottles are one of the safest options. They quickly are becoming the favorite among moms who want to feed their little ones safely. As the demand increases, glass bottle manufacturers are working on ways to make safer and shatter-free glass. Additionally you can purchase silicon sleeves for your baby's bottle, just as you use cases to protect your cell phone.

Experts say you can keep using your plastic bottles, but it is important to avoid overheating the plastic. Heat the milk in a glass bowl or on the stove, and then pour it into the bottle. If the plastic is scratched, toss it. All of these things cause the chemicals used in the production process to be released. Please do your homework before you purchase bottles for your little one.

CONCLUSION

For some of you this may be the beginning of your journey and for some you may have already been down this path before, regardless of where you are my hope is that you will continue to open yourself to learning. Attempt to read further on some of the issues that I have highlighted, I am certain you will learn something new and so much more. It was over a casual conversation with my eleven-year-old daughter today that I learned something new and very meaningful. She was learning about soap making and wound up finding out an interesting fact, upon further reading she learned that vegetable shortening was originally intended for use in soap manufacturing. It looked like lard, required no refrigeration and was cheaper to produce. It also proved great for cooking and baking that it ended up being used in food products instead. It was both exciting and somewhat of a personal victory in my day as I now know something that I didn't know yesterday. I do not use the product but instantly I related this little moment with my green living journey. There is still so much more I am yet to learn therefore my journey continues.

Go out and attempt to navigate your own path and make wise purchases that stem from an informed perspective. Be open, be excited, and focus on realistic changes that will work for you and your family. Remember that it is impossible to completely shield yourself and your family from all the harmful chemicals in this world but you can reduce your exposure. Little changes do yield big results that make a huge difference. It may be a little intimidating to try and tackle all of this at once. The key to success may be to phase out things one at a time. Start with the little things, like eating more organic foods. Then, replacing toxic cleaning products with safer options, buy local, and work your way up to some of the other things like making some of your own products if you are one of those people who love a DIY project. Talk to other mom's and share what you have learned. You have the power to do something and the opportunity to nurture the future today.